HEALING JOURNAL FOR AFTER MISCARRIAGE

Vicki Renz

Copyright © 2021 Vicki Renz

All rights reserved.

ISBN: 978-3-9823087-0-8

Honouring the memory of five beautiful angels who gave me the inspiration to start writing and creating

CONTENT

ACKNOWLEDGMENTS   *i*

ABOUT JOURNALING   1

ABOUT THE AUTHOR   187

ACKNOWLEDGMENTS

I am thankful for the healing journey that miscarriage took me on; opening up doors that I never knew existed. For the healers who have taught me the many skills I have and now use to guide others on their healing journeys. For the mentors who have encouraged and supported me to speak my voice, to become the person I am today. To my husband for being part of this journey with me and giving me the time to create my mission of support other women on their healing journey after miscarriage.

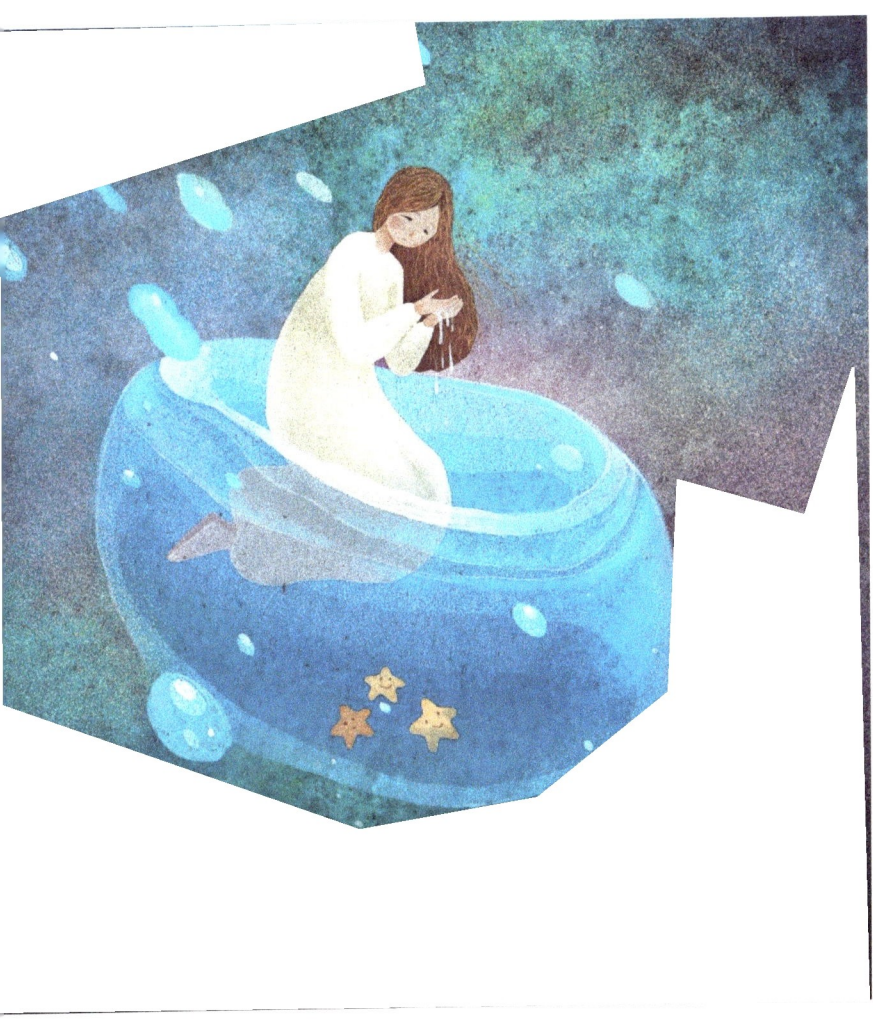

ABOUT JOURNALING

Journaling as an outlet

Journaling is a soul nourishing outlet for our thoughts, feelings and emotions. It is a safe space for us to talk with ourselves through the written word. Allowing us to pour our hearts out, letting our emotions flow out onto the page.

Journaling helps us to talk things through with ourselves, like a deep and meaningful one-to-one conversation. Journaling helps us to process and release.

Journaling as a healing technique

As Buddha said "the mind is everything; what you think you become". It can be all too easy to let our mind start running through an endless chitter chatter of negativity. After miscarriage we often wonder what we could have done differently, we wonder if it was our fault and it can go on and on. Our minds can be so unkind to us. If we allow the negative chatter to continue, we end up believing it about ourselves which can really eat away at our self-confidence.

Journaling can be used to turn this around. It can be used as a tool for turning the negative into the positive. Helping us to quieten the negativity down and feel better about ourselves. It is truly liberating when the positivity starts flowing, bringing more confidence and empowerment back into our lives.

Journaling Tips

Make journaling part of your morning and evening routine. Reserve time each day for focussing on journal time.

Free writing: firstly allow your thoughts and feelings to flow freely as you write. This is very therapeutic. Write until you are content and have released everything that was on your mind.

Express gratitude: write about what you are grateful for in your life. This brings in much positivity as you list out all of the good things. Some days are easier than others. Find at least three things that you are grateful for and write them down.

Positive affirmations: be kind to yourself. Speak to yourself as you would to your best friend. Write down positive statements about yourself, starting with "I am" at the beginning to make the statement present. Writing positive affirmations about yourself is a confidence boosting exercise. Write down at least three statements about yourself.

Visualisation: what do you want to have in your life? How do you visualise your life to be? Imagine the feeling how it would be if your life was like this now. That's the power of visualisation; we tell our brain that we already have this life and therefore bring it into being. This is based on the law of attraction. You can write statements in the form of gratitude for having these things in your life, even if they are not yet there, you are attracting them into being in your life.

HEALING JOURNAL FOR AFTER MISCARRIAGE

HEALING JOURNAL FOR AFTER MISCARRIAGE

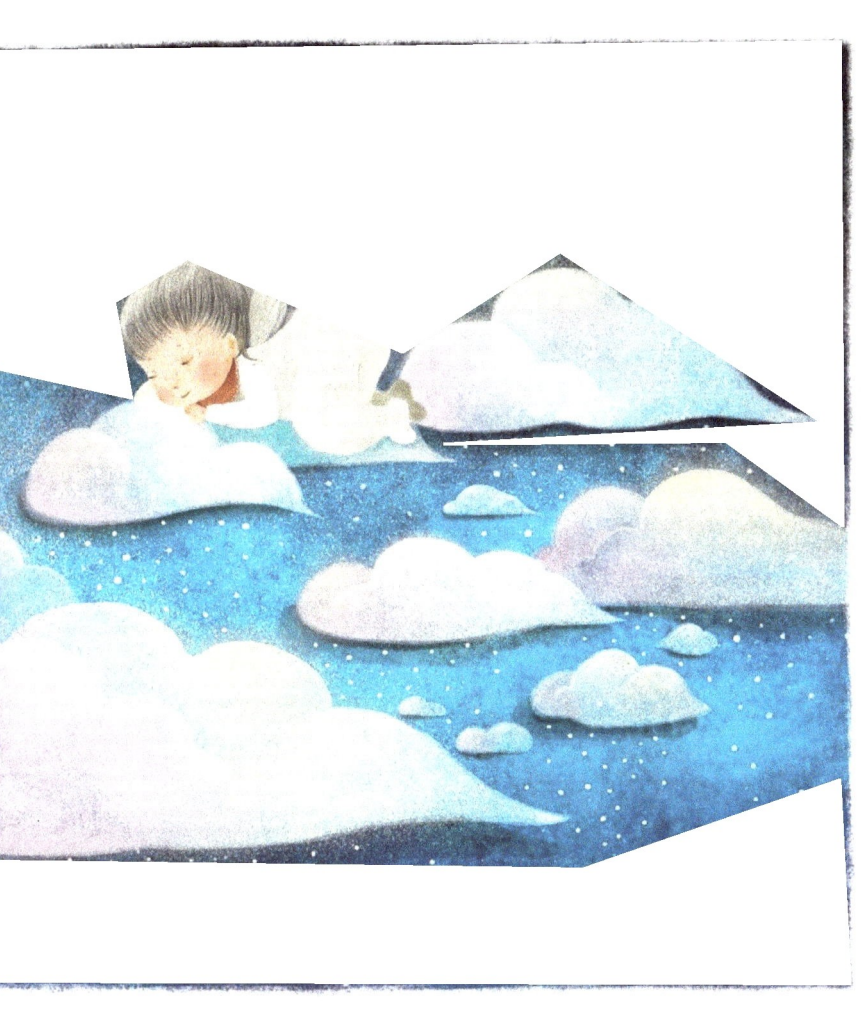

HEALING JOURNAL FOR AFTER MISCARRIAGE

HEALING JOURNAL FOR AFTER MISCARRIAGE

HEALING JOURNAL FOR AFTER MISCARRIAGE

HEALING JOURNAL FOR AFTER MISCARRIAGE

HEALING JOURNAL FOR AFTER MISCARRIAGE

HEALING JOURNAL FOR AFTER MISCARRIAGE

HEALING JOURNAL FOR AFTER MISCARRIAGE

HEALING JOURNAL FOR AFTER MISCARRIAGE

HEALING JOURNAL FOR AFTER MISCARRIAGE

HEALING JOURNAL FOR AFTER MISCARRIAGE

HEALING JOURNAL FOR AFTER MISCARRIAGE

HEALING JOURNAL FOR AFTER MISCARRIAGE

HEALING JOURNAL FOR AFTER MISCARRIAGE

HEALING JOURNAL FOR AFTER MISCARRIAGE

HEALING JOURNAL FOR AFTER MISCARRIAGE

HEALING JOURNAL FOR AFTER MISCARRIAGE

HEALING JOURNAL FOR AFTER MISCARRIAGE

HEALING JOURNAL FOR AFTER MISCARRIAGE

HEALING JOURNAL FOR AFTER MISCARRIAGE

HEALING JOURNAL FOR AFTER MISCARRIAGE

HEALING JOURNAL FOR AFTER MISCARRIAGE

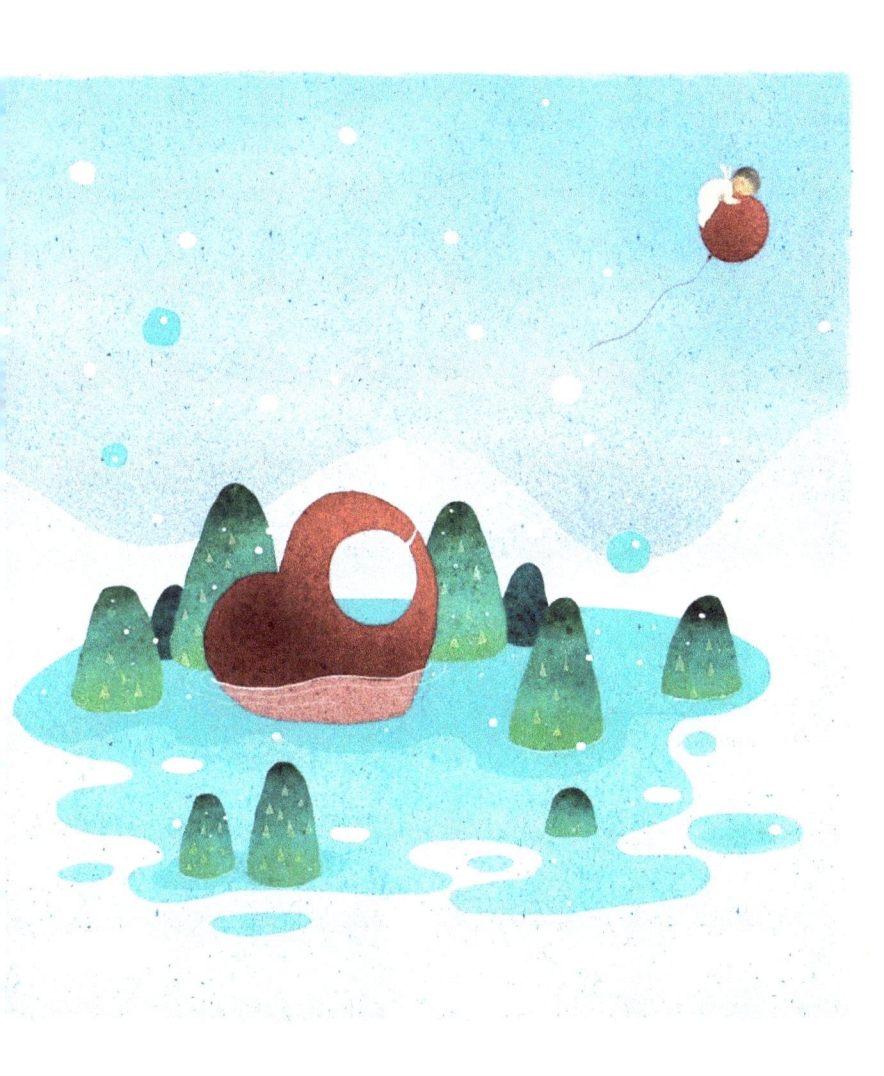

HEALING JOURNAL FOR AFTER MISCARRIAGE

HEALING JOURNAL FOR AFTER MISCARRIAGE

HEALING JOURNAL FOR AFTER MISCARRIAGE

HEALING JOURNAL FOR AFTER MISCARRIAGE

HEALING JOURNAL FOR AFTER MISCARRIAGE

HEALING JOURNAL FOR AFTER MISCARRIAGE

HEALING JOURNAL FOR AFTER MISCARRIAGE

HEALING JOURNAL FOR AFTER MISCARRIAGE

HEALING JOURNAL FOR AFTER MISCARRIAGE

HEALING JOURNAL FOR AFTER MISCARRIAGE

HEALING JOURNAL FOR AFTER MISCARRIAGE

HEALING JOURNAL FOR AFTER MISCARRIAGE

HEALING JOURNAL FOR AFTER MISCARRIAGE

HEALING JOURNAL FOR AFTER MISCARRIAGE

HEALING JOURNAL FOR AFTER MISCARRIAGE

HEALING JOURNAL FOR AFTER MISCARRIAGE

HEALING JOURNAL FOR AFTER MISCARRIAGE

HEALING JOURNAL FOR AFTER MISCARRIAGE

HEALING JOURNAL FOR AFTER MISCARRIAGE

HEALING JOURNAL FOR AFTER MISCARRIAGE

HEALING JOURNAL FOR AFTER MISCARRIAGE

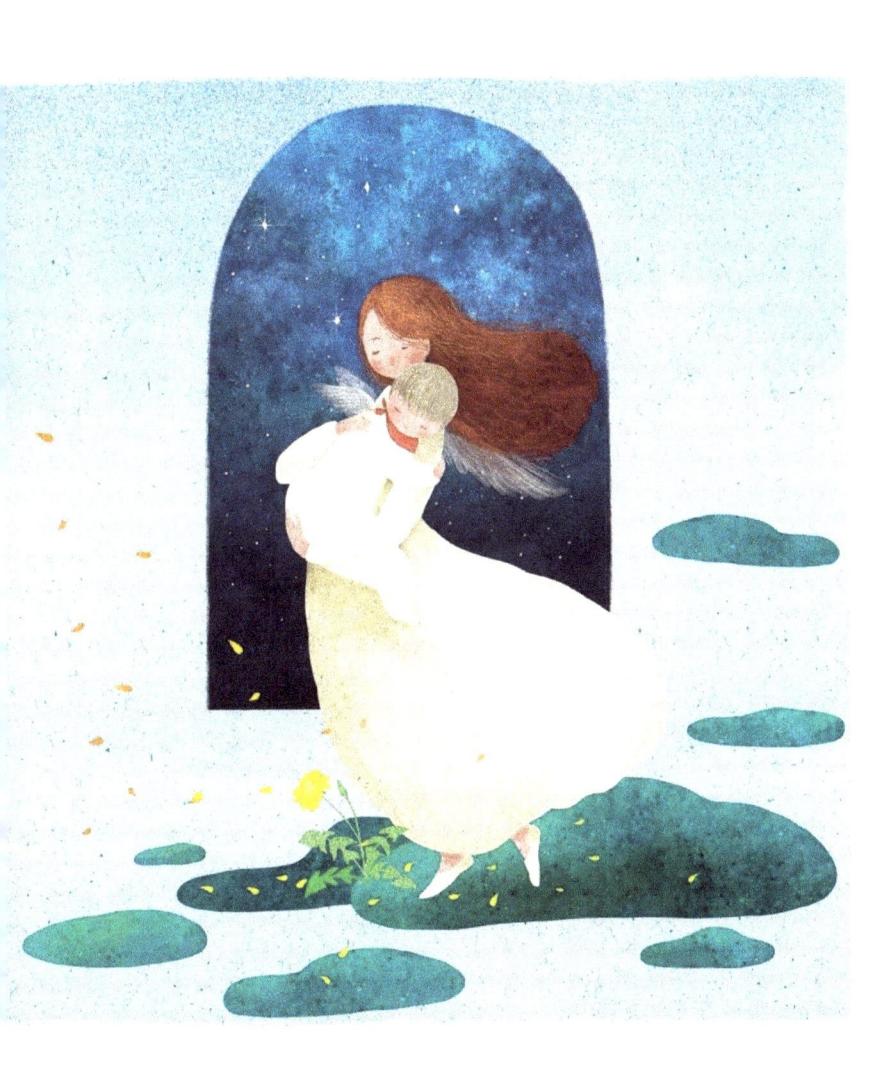

HEALING JOURNAL FOR AFTER MISCARRIAGE

HEALING JOURNAL FOR AFTER MISCARRIAGE

HEALING JOURNAL FOR AFTER MISCARRIAGE

HEALING JOURNAL FOR AFTER MISCARRIAGE

… HEALING JOURNAL FOR AFTER MISCARRIAGE

HEALING JOURNAL FOR AFTER MISCARRIAGE

HEALING JOURNAL FOR AFTER MISCARRIAGE

HEALING JOURNAL FOR AFTER MISCARRIAGE

HEALING JOURNAL FOR AFTER MISCARRIAGE

HEALING JOURNAL FOR AFTER MISCARRIAGE

HEALING JOURNAL FOR AFTER MISCARRIAGE

HEALING JOURNAL FOR AFTER MISCARRIAGE

HEALING JOURNAL FOR AFTER MISCARRIAGE

HEALING JOURNAL FOR AFTER MISCARRIAGE

HEALING JOURNAL FOR AFTER MISCARRIAGE

… HEALING JOURNAL FOR AFTER MISCARRIAGE

HEALING JOURNAL FOR AFTER MISCARRIAGE

HEALING JOURNAL FOR AFTER MISCARRIAGE

HEALING JOURNAL FOR AFTER MISCARRIAGE

HEALING JOURNAL FOR AFTER MISCARRIAGE

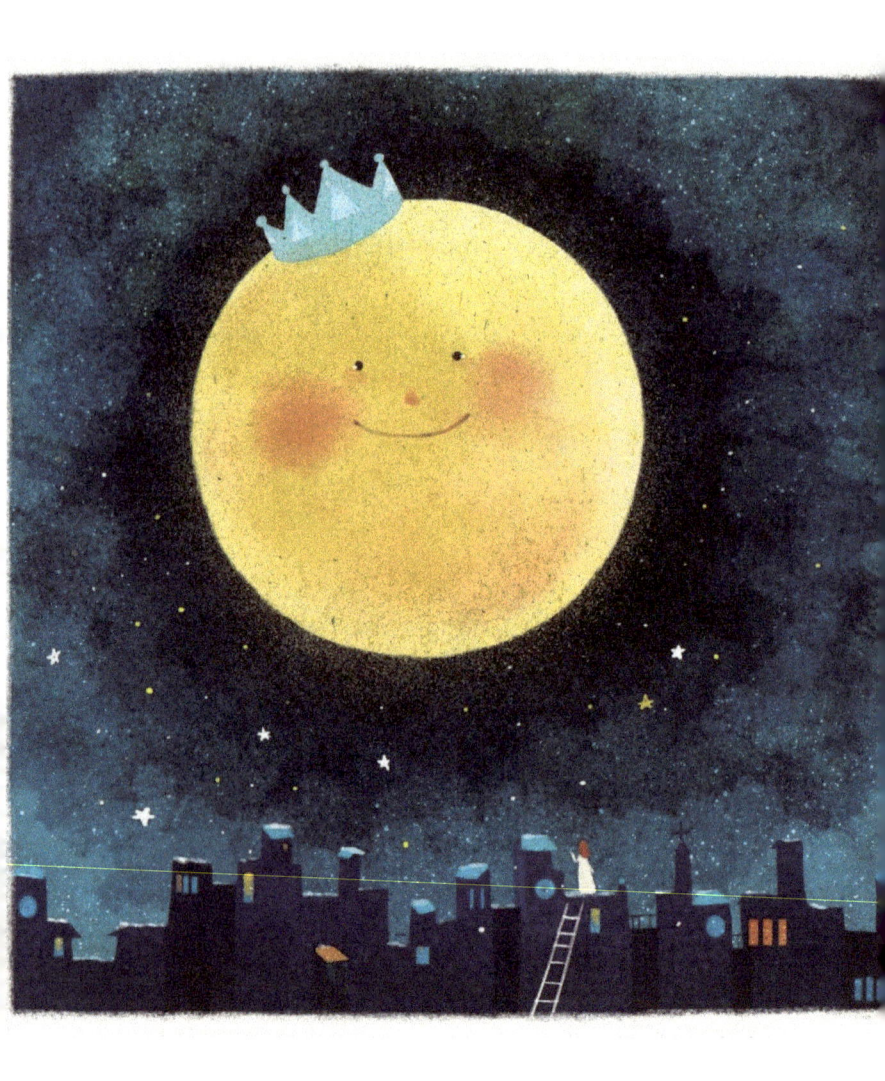

HEALING JOURNAL FOR AFTER MISCARRIAGE

HEALING JOURNAL FOR AFTER MISCARRIAGE

HEALING JOURNAL FOR AFTER MISCARRIAGE

HEALING JOURNAL FOR AFTER MISCARRIAGE

HEALING JOURNAL FOR AFTER MISCARRIAGE

HEALING JOURNAL FOR AFTER MISCARRIAGE

HEALING JOURNAL FOR AFTER MISCARRIAGE

HEALING JOURNAL FOR AFTER MISCARRIAGE

HEALING JOURNAL FOR AFTER MISCARRIAGE

HEALING JOURNAL FOR AFTER MISCARRIAGE

HEALING JOURNAL FOR AFTER MISCARRIAGE

HEALING JOURNAL FOR AFTER MISCARRIAGE

HEALING JOURNAL FOR AFTER MISCARRIAGE

HEALING JOURNAL FOR AFTER MISCARRIAGE

HEALING JOURNAL FOR AFTER MISCARRIAGE

HEALING JOURNAL FOR AFTER MISCARRIAGE

… HEALING JOURNAL FOR AFTER MISCARRIAGE

HEALING JOURNAL FOR AFTER MISCARRIAGE

HEALING JOURNAL FOR AFTER MISCARRIAGE

HEALING JOURNAL FOR AFTER MISCARRIAGE

HEALING JOURNAL FOR AFTER MISCARRIAGE

HEALING JOURNAL FOR AFTER MISCARRIAGE

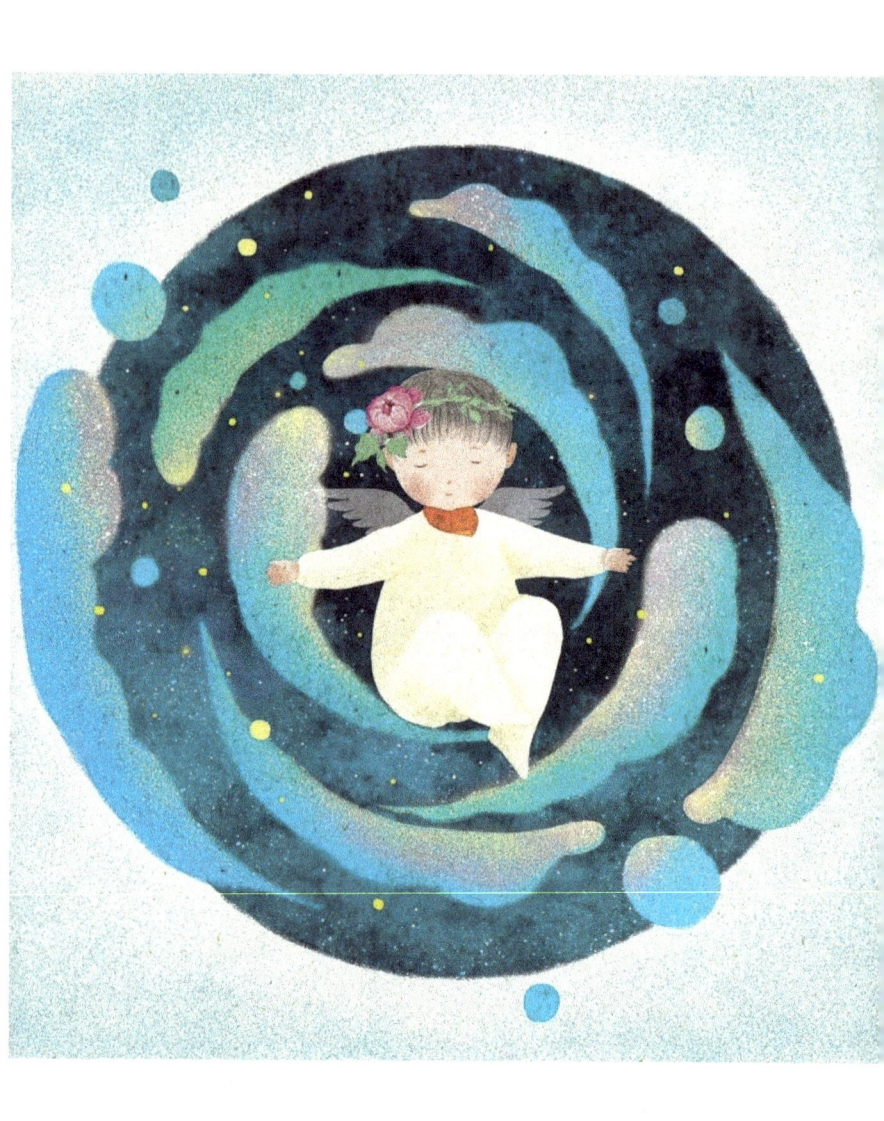

HEALING JOURNAL FOR AFTER MISCARRIAGE

— HEALING JOURNAL FOR AFTER MISCARRIAGE —

HEALING JOURNAL FOR AFTER MISCARRIAGE

HEALING JOURNAL FOR AFTER MISCARRIAGE

HEALING JOURNAL FOR AFTER MISCARRIAGE

HEALING JOURNAL FOR AFTER MISCARRIAGE

HEALING JOURNAL FOR AFTER MISCARRIAGE

HEALING JOURNAL FOR AFTER MISCARRIAGE

HEALING JOURNAL FOR AFTER MISCARRIAGE

HEALING JOURNAL FOR AFTER MISCARRIAGE

HEALING JOURNAL FOR AFTER MISCARRIAGE

HEALING JOURNAL FOR AFTER MISCARRIAGE

HEALING JOURNAL FOR AFTER MISCARRIAGE

HEALING JOURNAL FOR AFTER MISCARRIAGE

HEALING JOURNAL FOR AFTER MISCARRIAGE

HEALING JOURNAL FOR AFTER MISCARRIAGE

HEALING JOURNAL FOR AFTER MISCARRIAGE

HEALING JOURNAL FOR AFTER MISCARRIAGE

HEALING JOURNAL FOR AFTER MISCARRIAGE

HEALING JOURNAL FOR AFTER MISCARRIAGE

HEALING JOURNAL FOR AFTER MISCARRIAGE

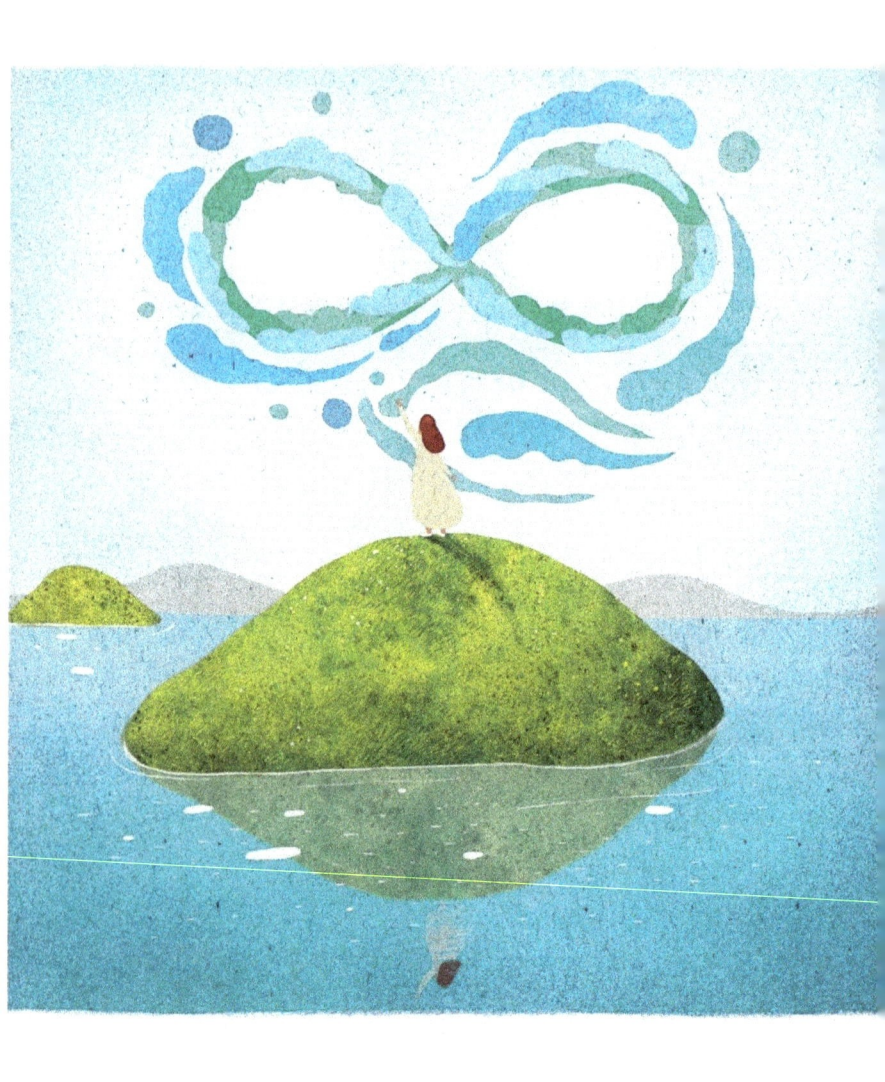

HEALING JOURNAL FOR AFTER MISCARRIAGE

HEALING JOURNAL FOR AFTER MISCARRIAGE

HEALING JOURNAL FOR AFTER MISCARRIAGE

HEALING JOURNAL FOR AFTER MISCARRIAGE

HEALING JOURNAL FOR AFTER MISCARRIAGE

HEALING JOURNAL FOR AFTER MISCARRIAGE

HEALING JOURNAL FOR AFTER MISCARRIAGE

HEALING JOURNAL FOR AFTER MISCARRIAGE

HEALING JOURNAL FOR AFTER MISCARRIAGE

HEALING JOURNAL FOR AFTER MISCARRIAGE

HEALING JOURNAL FOR AFTER MISCARRIAGE

HEALING JOURNAL FOR AFTER MISCARRIAGE

HEALING JOURNAL FOR AFTER MISCARRIAGE

HEALING JOURNAL FOR AFTER MISCARRIAGE

HEALING JOURNAL FOR AFTER MISCARRIAGE

HEALING JOURNAL FOR AFTER MISCARRIAGE

HEALING JOURNAL FOR AFTER MISCARRIAGE

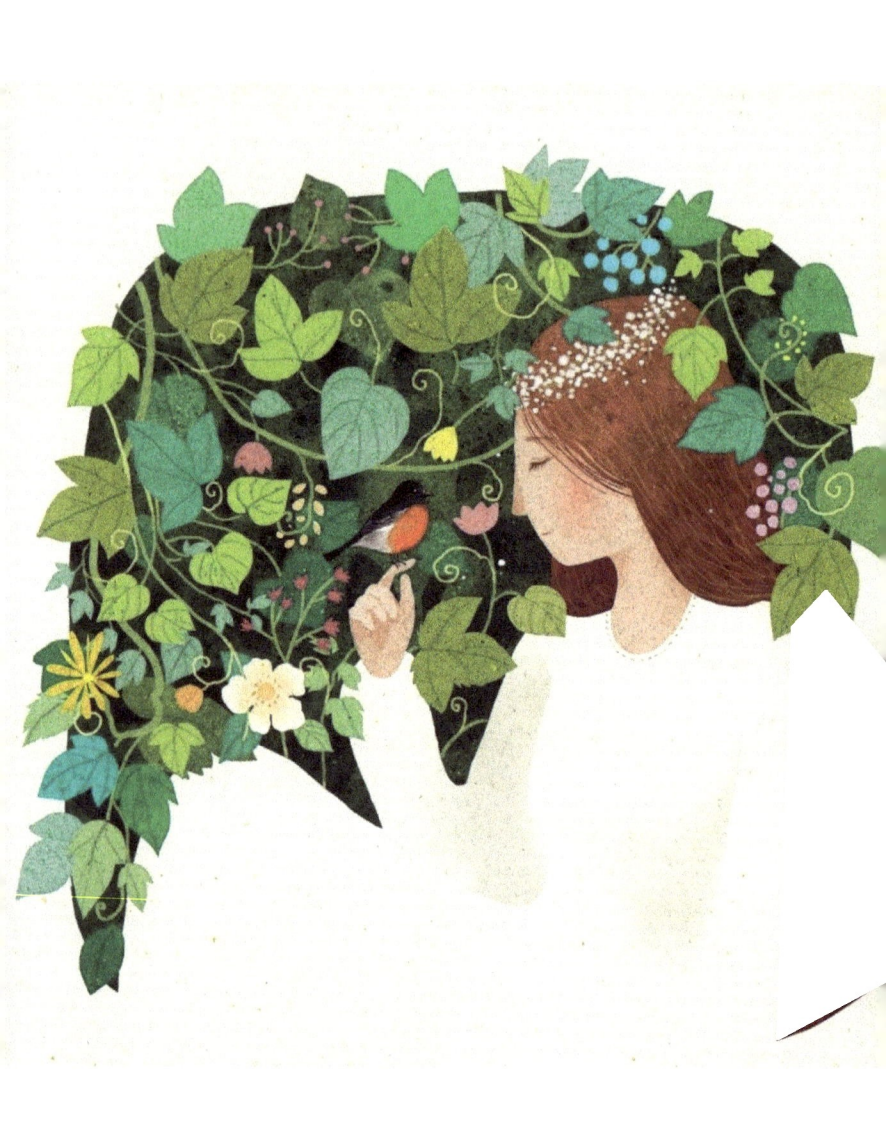

HEALING JOURNAL FOR AFTER MISCARRIAGE

HEALING JOURNAL FOR AFTER MISCARRIAGE

HEALING JOURNAL FOR AFTER MISCARRIAGE

HEALING JOURNAL FOR AFTER MISCARRIAGE

HEALING JOURNAL FOR AFTER MISCARRIAGE

HEALING JOURNAL FOR AFTER MISCARRIAGE

HEALING JOURNAL FOR AFTER MISCARRIAGE

HEALING JOURNAL FOR AFTER MISCARRIAGE

HEALING JOURNAL FOR AFTER MISCARRIAGE

HEALING JOURNAL FOR AFTER MISCARRIAGE

HEALING JOURNAL FOR AFTER MISCARRIAGE

HEALING JOURNAL FOR AFTER MISCARRIAGE

HEALING JOURNAL FOR AFTER MISCARRIAGE

HEALING JOURNAL FOR AFTER MISCARRIAGE

HEALING JOURNAL FOR AFTER MISCARRIAGE

HEALING JOURNAL FOR AFTER MISCARRIAGE

HEALING JOURNAL FOR AFTER MISCARRIAGE

HEALING JOURNAL FOR AFTER MISCARRIAGE

HEALING JOURNAL FOR AFTER MISCARRIAGE

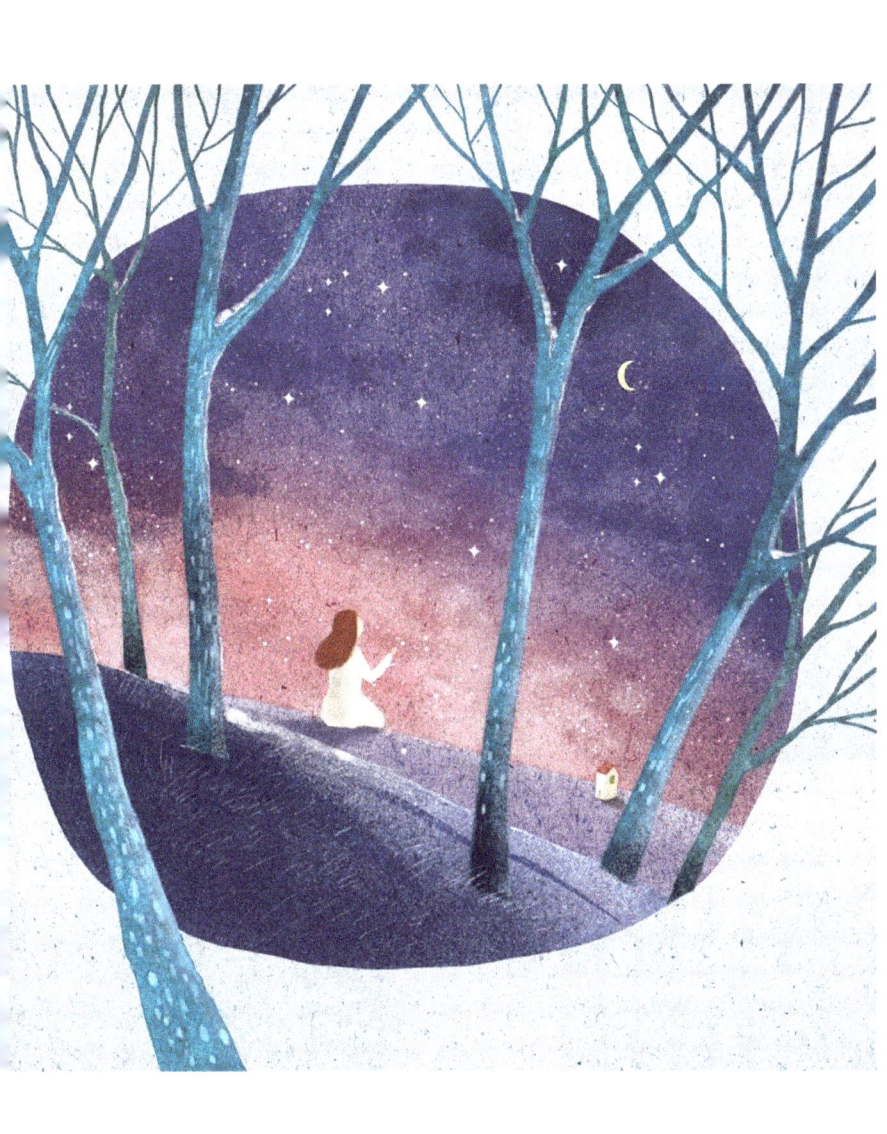

HEALING JOURNAL FOR AFTER MISCARRIAGE

HEALING JOURNAL FOR AFTER MISCARRIAGE

HEALING JOURNAL FOR AFTER MISCARRIAGE

HEALING JOURNAL FOR AFTER MISCARRIAGE

HEALING JOURNAL FOR AFTER MISCARRIAGE

HEALING JOURNAL FOR AFTER MISCARRIAGE

HEALING JOURNAL FOR AFTER MISCARRIAGE

HEALING JOURNAL FOR AFTER MISCARRIAGE

HEALING JOURNAL FOR AFTER MISCARRIAGE

HEALING JOURNAL FOR AFTER MISCARRIAGE

HEALING JOURNAL FOR AFTER MISCARRIAGE

HEALING JOURNAL FOR AFTER MISCARRIAGE

HEALING JOURNAL FOR AFTER MISCARRIAGE

HEALING JOURNAL FOR AFTER MISCARRIAGE

HEALING JOURNAL FOR AFTER MISCARRIAGE

… HEALING JOURNAL FOR AFTER MISCARRIAGE

HEALING JOURNAL FOR AFTER MISCARRIAGE

HEALING JOURNAL FOR AFTER MISCARRIAGE

ABOUT THE AUTHOR

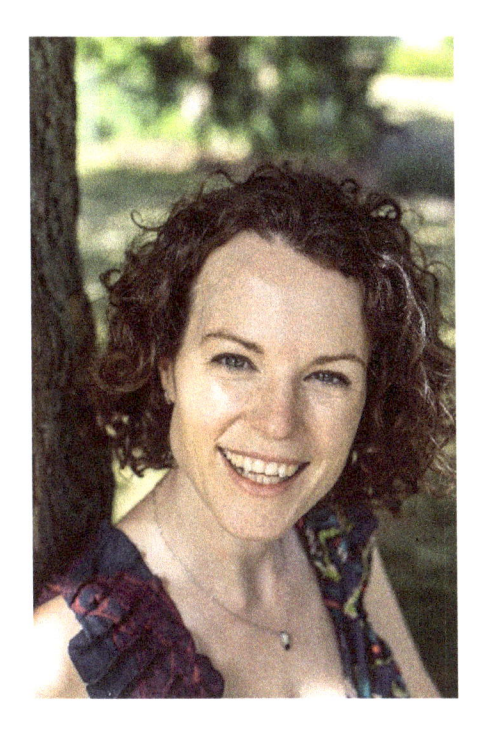

Vicki Renz, mother to two boys and recurrent miscarriage survivor, is founder and director of Oh My Mama Body, the specialist portal for women (ohmymamabody.com).

The empathy that exudes from Oh My Mama Body makes Vicki an honest source that thousands of women trust. After going through the traumatic experience of multiple miscarriages, Vicki embarked on a deep study of healing techniques.

Vicki mastered healing techniques and developed her unique Pathway to Wholeness coaching programme to help others with their journeys. Like a guiding light, Vicki coaches women through their journey from pain and grief through to acceptance, wholeness and empowerment.

If you feel like you are caught up in a web of emotions and feeling like half the person you were before. Are you just trying to hold it together and would like guidance on how to grow your inner-strength again, visit Vicki's transformational coaching programme.

Sometimes it just takes an outside perspective to open up the pathway to moving forward. Vicki understands the depth of your emotions and provides a pathway to move you through the cycle of grief to becoming whole and empowered again.

Follow the link below for all of Vicki's healing after miscarriage supportive resources:

https://ohmymamabody.com/healing-after-miscarriage/

CPSIA information can be obtained
at www.ICGtesting.com
Printed in the USA
LVHW070101010723
751124LV00014B/153